Good Night

YOUR HOLISTIC GUIDE
TO THE BEST SLEEP
OF YOUR LIFE

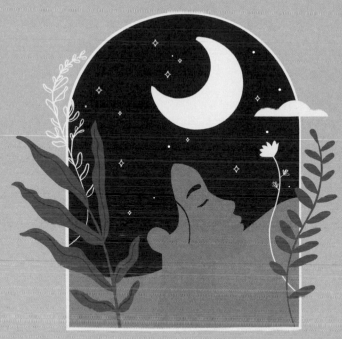

Good Night

YOUR HOLISTIC GUIDE TO
THE BEST SLEEP OF YOUR LIFE

Julia Blohberger and Roos Neeter

Illustrations by Roel Steenbergen

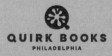

QUIRK BOOKS

PHILADELPHIA

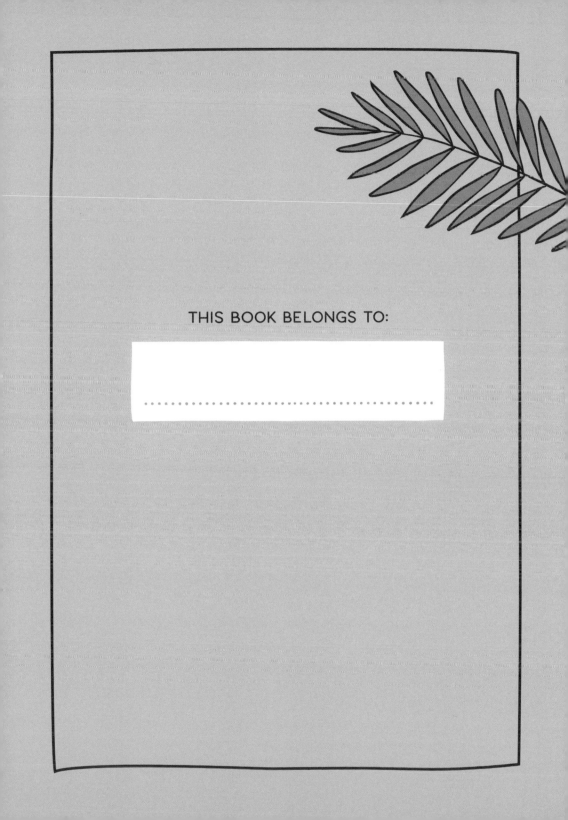

THIS BOOK BELONGS TO:

....

Contents

Let's Go to Bed

Why is a good night's rest so elusive for so many?

Problems with sleep often arise from some form of stress. Most of us experience stress on a daily basis in some area of our lives: work, family, relationships, health, bills, and more. But our evolving lifestyles have increased our daily dose of stress to sometimes unmanageable levels. Many of us are working more than ever and spending more time indoors, where we stare at screens and scroll through various news and social media platforms for hours on end. It's no wonder so many of us struggle with sleep!

Sleeplessness is rarely an isolated issue, though. If you're having a hard time going to bed and staying asleep, your body and mind are likely experiencing other issues, including indigestion, anxiety, and aches and pains. This is your body's way of saying, "Help! I'm overstressed and need a break!" But the only way to fully recharge and rebuild energy is to sleep. If you're incapable of achieving deep, restful sleep, the sleep-stress cycle continues until you either burn out or check out.

The good news is that there are plenty of things you can do to get more rest, especially if you adopt a holistic approach to solving your sleep issues. This book provides plenty of tips and tricks to achieve deep and restful sleep, which will give you more energy to face the day, focus, process information, and manage your stress. We know that combing through the massive amounts of sleep research available today is already enough to make you tired, so we've done that hard work for you. You don't need to be a practitioner of Ayurveda to follow our tips—we think you'll find that much of our advice is intuitive, logical, and easy to apply. However, it helps to understand that we see sleep as a time to connect to a universal power source, which allows you to mentally process all the experiences of your day and live with a fresh and open mind. That universal power source allows you to be attuned not only to yourself but to the rest of the world.

We recommend that you spend at least a week absorbing the information in this book, following the journal prompts, and tracking your sleep without making any adjustments. After that, we recommend implementing whichever of our practices, rituals, and techniques make sense for you and tracking your progress in the twenty-one day tracker at the end of this book. This will give you insight into how your sleep is impacted by your lifestyle choices and stress levels so you can make adjustments along the way and afterward.

A final note: throughout this book, we will refer to five elements: **earth, water, fire, wind,** and **space**. In Ayurveda, these elements carry specific inherent qualities:

* Qualities of earth: heaviness and slowness

* Qualities of water: flowing and softness

* Qualities of fire: heat and transformation

* Qualities of wind: movement and dryness

* Qualities of space: subtleness and lightness

Without further ado, let's get into bed.

LOVE, JULIA & ROOS

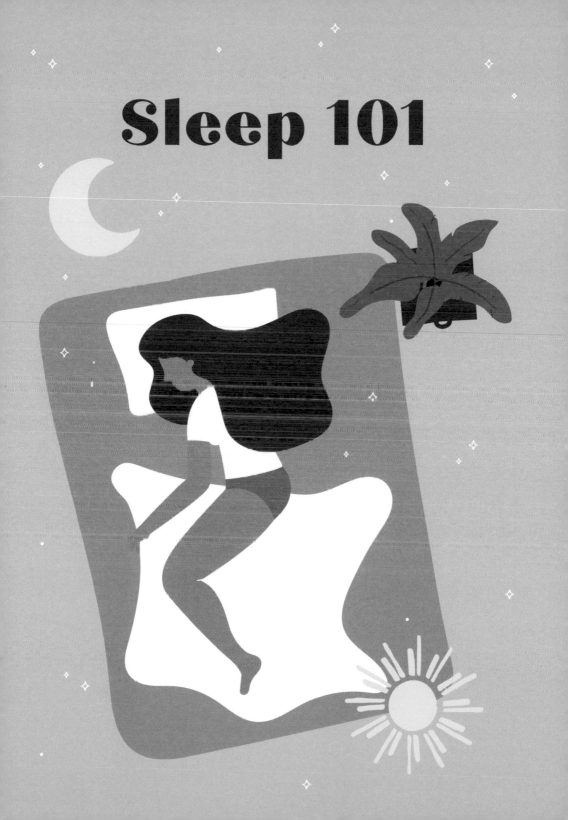

Sleep 101

Before we dive into life hacks and sleep remedies, we need to go over the basics. This section will help you understand the four stages of sleep and how your environment impacts your sleep. This section is more informational than functional, though we do include a few tips throughout to improve your sleep space. Let's shine a (night) light on some need-to-know sleep information!

The Four Stages
of Sleep

Sleep works in a four-stage cycle. The first three stages are the quiet sleep or NREM (non–rapid eye movement) stages. The fourth stage is the active sleep or REM (rapid eye movement) stage. One cycle takes about 90 to 120 minutes to complete, and your body goes through the cycle several times each night.

These four stages impact the biological processes that control your body temperature, cellular function, muscle function, and breathing. At the same time, the sleep cycle allows your brain to organize, rearrange, and store memories.

Here's how the four stages work, according to our current understanding of sleep science:

1   **NREM stage 1:** In this stage, your body shifts from wakefulness into sleep. Your brain activity, heartbeat, eye movement, muscle tension, and breathing all relax and slow down.

2   **NREM stage 2:** In this stage, your eye movement stops, your body temperature drops, and your heart rate continues to slow. You're barely aware of your surroundings.

3   **NREM stage 3:** In this stage, you're in such deep sleep that surrounding noises or activities might not even wake you up. It is in this stage that your body repairs itself. Your muscles are fully relaxed and your breathing is slow.

4   **REM stage:** This is also known as the dream stage. Your brain activity picks up again but your body stays completely relaxed. This is the phase when your dreams are most vivid and your body is temporarily paralyzed to prevent you from physically

reacting to your dreams. Repair, deep restoration, and resetting of the brain occur in this stage.

After one complete cycle, many people wake up briefly but remain unaware before the cycle begins again. If you often feel sluggish in the morning and tired throughout the day, it's possible you're not sleeping long enough for your body to complete multiple cycles.

Early to Bed, Early to Rise, Makes a (Wo)Man Healthy, Wealthy, and Wise

Ayurveda encourages us to be in touch with our natural circadian rhythms. The evening—from about 6 p.m. to 10 p.m.—is when we (should) naturally slow down. Our focus should be on unwinding from the day and leaving work and noise behind (yes, that includes the news and social media). This is the best way to feel more relaxed and to achieve a state of sleepiness, which is an important factor in a good night's rest.

The perfect time to take a boat to dreamland is 10 p.m. After that, our inner fire starts rising again, which means we might get hungry for a snack, feel inspired to do some work that's waiting for us, or binge a TV show. This urge is a spark of light from the fire element within you. It can be tempting to give into this urge, but if you do, it'll be very difficult to get enough quality sleep by the time you need to wake up the next day.

It's important to be *in bed* before your fire starts burning so you can use it to process all the mental impressions from your day during sleep. That fire will help you digest experiences, transform them into memories, and discard what you don't need, leaving you with a clean slate for a brand-new day.

Your body is clever and knows just what to do. You just need to listen to it and follow its natural rhythms.

Safe and Heavy

In order to fall asleep, we need to allow a sense of heaviness to take over our bodies and give in to the downward force of the earth. (That's why it's called "falling" asleep!) But before we can fall, we have to *feel safe*. Feeling nervous or anxious prevents our bodies from surrendering to that heaviness because we don't feel safe. If our minds are fragile, our bodies retain a quality of lightness that makes it hard for that heaviness to set in.

If you're having trouble generating a sense of heaviness, you can create it externally. A heavy or weighted blanket is a great way to do this; the weight of the blanket gives your mind a sense of safety, of being held and nurtured. Just make sure to choose a well-ventilated blanket!

A Mattress Made in Heaven

If you regularly notice yourself tossing and turning overnight or waking up with shoulder or back pain, you might be picking up on signs that you and your mattress are not a match made in heaven.

The quality of your mattress has a huge effect on your physical well-being and, therefore, your ability to get a good night's rest. This doesn't necessarily mean you need to buy an expensive mattress (though we do recommend spending as much as your budget allows on a quality one). You just have to take some time to understand your needs.

There are many types of mattresses available: hard as a brick, soft and foamy, in-between, and even undulating (remember waterbeds?). If you find yourself changing positions frequently throughout the night and waking up with achy body parts, we recommend that you go to a physical mattress store and test-drive different types of mattresses. There are also online retailers that will ship a mattress to you and let you try it out for a period of time. If you don't like it, you can return it!

If you sleep with a partner who has different mattress needs, consider investing in an adjustable bed that's the width of a traditional king-sized bed but contains two twin mattresses, each of which can be customized to your individual needs.

The perfect mattress is out there waiting for you!

Say No to Screens

We all know this but it's worth saying again: don't bring your electronic devices to bed!

Yep, it's a bummer but if you're truly serious about improving your sleep hygiene, this has to be on your list. It's tough to let go of a bedtime screen habit, but scrolling through your phone or watching TV keeps you up, plain and simple. Devices keep your mind active at a time when it needs to slow down and prepare for heaviness. Sometimes screen time can seem harmless, especially if you're enjoying a favorite TV show, but your brain needs to fall asleep before your body can—and it can't if you're keeping it awake.

There has been lots of research conducted about blue light—a type of light emitted from electronic devices—and how devices that emit blue light can disrupt your natural sleep cycle. While theories about blue light impacting your vision are widely disputed, laboratory studies show that blue light decreases your melatonin levels. Melatonin is a hormone made in the pineal gland that helps set the time of your internal clock. Getting enough sunlight during the day and decreasing blue light in the evening supports your circadian rhythms, allowing you to naturally feel sleepy at the end of the day.

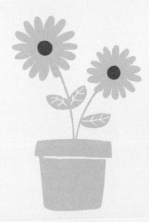

OBSERVE YOUR SLEEP SPACE.
WHAT IS THE QUALITY OF THE LIGHT?
IS IT CONDUCIVE TO SLEEPINESS?
ARE THERE TECHNOLOGICAL DEVICES IN THE ROOM
THAT CAN BE RELOCATED TO ANOTHER ROOM?

USE THIS SPACE TO REFLECT ON HOW YOU CAN IMPROVE YOUR SLEEP SPACE.

Bedroom Prana

In Sanskrit, *prana* means "breath." As a concept in Ayurveda, prana is the energy that drives life. It's a complex idea and we could write a whole book about it, but we don't want to get too far into the weeds in the context of this book. Let's focus on the prana of your physical sleep space, which has an impact on your body, mind, and soul—and, therefore, your ability to rest.

Indoor plants are more popular than ever, and we personally love them! They clean the air and have an instant calming effect on your mind. Most feng shui experts tout their restorative qualities, but they don't account for the fact that some plants also release larger quantities of carbon dioxide at night as a by-product of cellular respiration. This affects our breathing patterns during a time when our bodies naturally want to take in more oxygen. If you toss and turn a lot, you might be sharing your space with too many green friends. We spend a huge portion of our lives in our bedrooms, so the power of the plants in our sleep space shouldn't be underestimated.

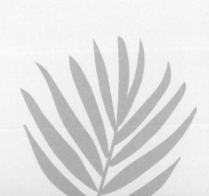

If you're intent on keeping plants in your sleep space, prioritize ones that release oxygen at night, including cacti, bromeliads, and some succulents. This category includes:

* Angel wings cactus

* African milk tree

* Saguaro cactus

* Blushing bromeliad

* Scarlet star bromeliad

* Aloe vera

* Spider plant

* Snake plant

* Peace lily

If you have pets in your home, make sure that your plants are compatible with them as well as with your sleep environment.

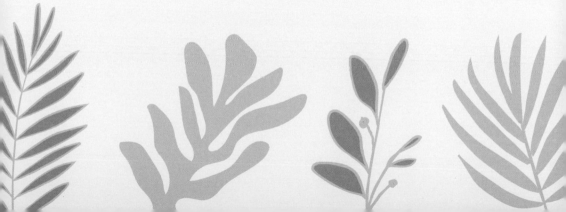

THIS IS YOUR SPACE TO REFLECT ON YOUR
RELATIONSHIP WITH SLEEP.
ARE YOU HAPPY WITH THE QUALITY AND LENGTH
OF YOUR SLEEP LATELY?

WHAT IS HOLDING YOU BACK FROM YOUR IDEAL SLEEP EXPERIENCE?
WHAT CHANGES WOULD YOU LIKE TO MAKE?

Week One Tracker

	MONDAY	TUESDAY	WEDNESDAY
TIME OF LAST MEAL			
TIME OF LAST CAFFEINE INTAKE			
TIME OF LAST ALCOHOL INTAKE			
TIME OF LAST WATER INTAKE			
SLEEP RITUALS			
SLEEP AIDS TAKEN			
TIME IN BED			
TIME YOU FELL ASLEEP			
DID YOU WAKE DURING THE NIGHT? (Y/N)			
MINUTES AWAKE			
NUMBER OF BATHROOM VISITS			
FINAL WAKE-UP TIME			
NIGHTMARES (Y/N)			
TOTAL HOURS OF SLEEP			
RESTED FEELING (1-10)			

We encourage you to write directly in this book! But if you'd like to track your sleep for longer than a week to spend more time studying your sleep patterns, then we suggest you photocopy the tracker as many times as you need.

THURSDAY	FRIDAY	SATURDAY	SUNDAY

Surrender to Rest

We (Julia and Roos) live in a Western society, so we understand deeply how the severe chronic stress of a Western lifestyle can impact your health and affect your sleep. There's the pressure to do well at work or school, to present yourself in a certain light on social media, and to handle all the big and small tasks of daily life. If you let all that pressure take over, it can be pretty intense. It is for many people.

Widespread access to computers is a new development within the scope of human history (and even more recent in Earth's whole history).

We are bombarded with more information than our brains can process, leaving us feeling overstimulated and anxious. This is why self-care is so important. No, not the kind of self-care where you purchase a lot of luxury skincare products (though we love a nice cream!). We're talking about protecting yourself against the chaos of the world so that you can engage with it in your own time, and rest to recover when you need to.

Oil Up

In Sanskrit, the word *sneha* means both "oil" and "love." That association explains why getting a massage can feel like the greatest act of self-love!

We love getting massages but let's face it: we don't all have the time and funds to get them regularly. That's why we recommend self-massaging. It's a great tool in your self-care and sleep-care toolkit, and you don't have to do more than buy a bottle of oil. (Not from the food section of your local grocery store, mind you. Select oil from the bath and body section or visit a health and beauty store.)

Making self-massage a part of your regular routine is a lovely way to step out of the rat race and soothe your parasympathetic nervous system, which controls rest and digestion. Oil is nourishing, grounding, and soothing. By massaging it onto your skin, you can climb out of mental traps and ground yourself in your body and physical surroundings.

Applying oil feels like a loving hug, which is a beautiful way to induce sleep. You can do this routine before showering or bathing at night. If you notice that showering before bedtime wakes you up, try showering as early in the evening as possible. You can also keep the oil on and wash it off the next morning, though some bedsheets might not take kindly to it!

There are many different kinds of oils, so we won't recommend one in particular. Let your nose and skin guide you. If an oil is too strong, your nose will tell you. If it's too viscous and doesn't absorb well, your skin will tell you. It's all up to your personal preferences.

Rinse Away
Your Worries

An evening bath or shower can have a tremendously beneficial effect on the quality of your sleep. It rids your physical body of dirt and cleanses your mind, energy, and spirit, allowing you to rinse off anything from the day that doesn't serve you.

Taking a warm bath one to two hours before bedtime, for as little as ten minutes, will help you drift off into la-la land by increasing your blood circulation and regulating your body temperature. This is especially important if you deal with restless limbs or feel too hot or cold as you're dozing off.

If you're used to taking a quick shower in the morning, consider switching to evening baths or showers as part of your sleep-care practice. A bath is a beautiful end-of-day ritual and a great way to replace screen time.

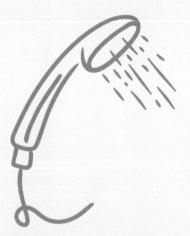

TAKE AN EVENING BATH OR SHOWER AND REFLECT ON IT
THE NEXT DAY. HOW DID IT MAKE YOU FEEL?
WERE YOU ABLE TO "RINSE OFF" YOUR TROUBLES?
DID IT POSITIVELY IMPACT YOUR SLEEP?

Five-Minute Foot Bath

Still resistant to bathing or showering in the evening? No worries, we've got you covered. A warm foot bath before bedtime is the next best thing and will do wonders for your mental health. A foot bath is also great if you're tight on time or simply don't have the energy to take a full bath. Just let your gorgeous feet rest in a warm water bath with some essential oil. We love rose and lavender oils for this.

To turn a foot bath into a sleep ritual:

* Place your feet in a bathtub or wide basin filled with warm water.

* Set a timer for five to ten minutes.

* Sit in a comfortable position with your spine upright and your shoulders relaxed.

* Close your eyes.

* Notice the feel of the water on your skin, the temperature, and any other sensations.

* Take a deep breath and send that breath all the way down to your feet as you exhale.

Once your alarm goes off, dry your feet and massage them with oil or your favorite nourishing cream.

The Foot-Body Connection

If you don't have time to oil your entire body before bed, focus solely on your feet. Our feet are often overlooked when it comes to self-care but they contain many pressure points and need regular attention. By massaging your feet with sesame, lavender, or almond oil, you can activate these points, which enhances relaxation—the key to a good night's sleep.

Your feet are the farthest body parts from your head so by giving them some extra love and attention you actively pull focus away from the mind and into your body.

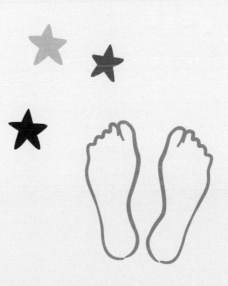

Legs Up

Practicing yoga promotes better and longer sleep. If a regular yoga class doesn't fit into your schedule, here's a simple pose you can do. This is a powerful restorative pose that not only helps you deeply relax your body but also calms your nervous system and mind. This pose can be practiced before sleep or if you wake up in the middle of the night.

* Lie down on your bed perpendicular to your headboard or the wall with your head resting on a comfortable pillow.

* Shimmy your hips as close to the headboard or wall as possible. As you're doing this, walk your feet up the headboard or wall until they are above your hips and the backs of your legs are resting against the wall. It's okay for your knees to be slightly bent. Keep your lower back on the mattress.

* If you have a lavender eye pillow, lay it over your closed eyes. Rest your arms on your belly or next to your body.

* Focus on your breath. Inhale and exhale until you establish a regular rhythm. If your mind is very active then extend your exhalations as long as possible.

* Remain in this position for up to twenty minutes.

Quick Fix for Twitchy Eyes

You're lying in your bed with your eyes closed but you can still feel them twitching. Sound familiar?

This might be an issue with your eyelids, which are unable to join your eyeballs in their relaxed and comfortable state. From a holistic perspective, this can mean that your wind element is too high, which causes too much movement in your body.

To calm your overactive eyelids, place an eye pillow on top of them, inviting them to relax and calm down. These little eye pillows are often filled with rice or flaxseeds and scented with lavender to enhance relaxation. You can purchase these online or at health and beauty stores.

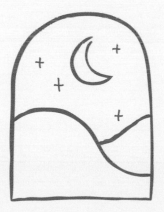

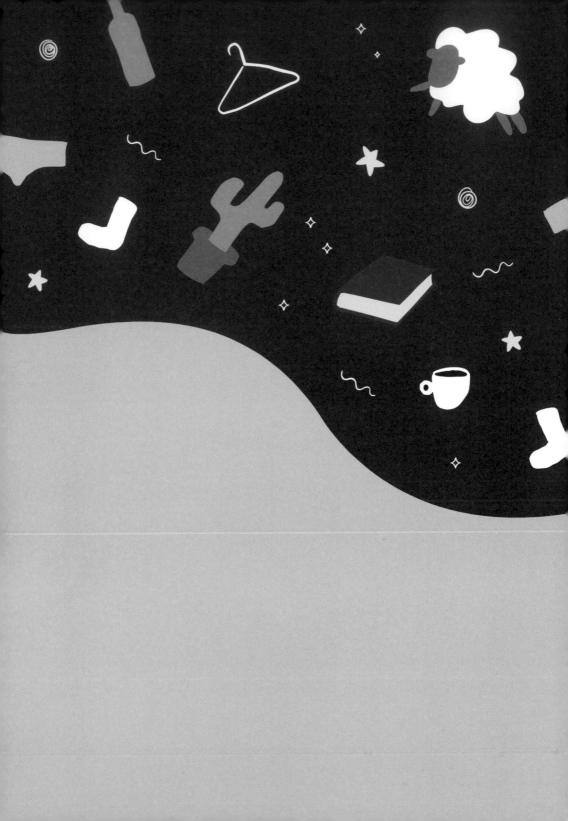

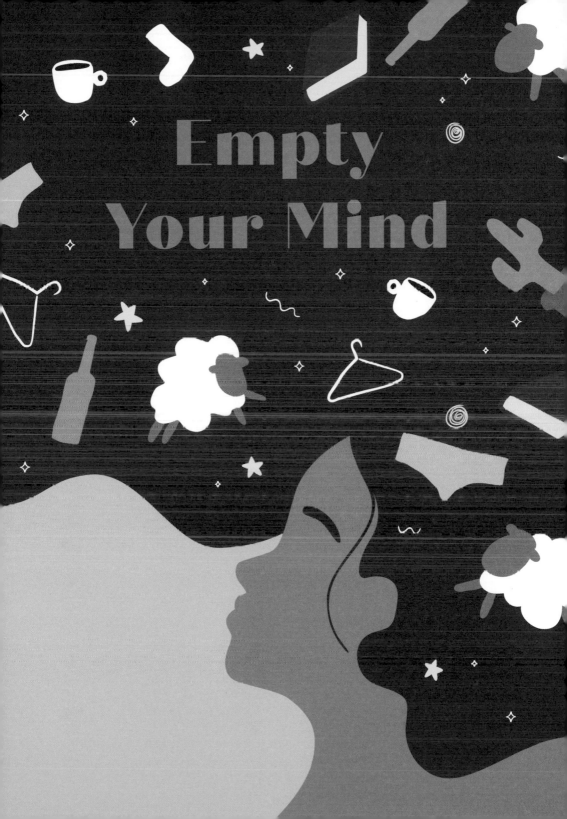

These days, modern conveniences have made it so we can do as little physical work as possible and still maintain a high quality of life. This allows us to focus more on our jobs and ourselves, which seems positive but in reality can be a double-edged sword.

In yoga, we are taught that living from the heart helps you achieve awareness but living from the mind increases your ego. When your ego grows, your point of view narrows, which cuts you off from the flow of life—especially its nonmaterial dimensions. When you lose touch with the outside world, it can be hard to maintain perspective, which can lead you to feel more easily overwhelmed and depleted.

Our minds—and egos—are working over-time. Clearing space in your mind is a good first step to achieving the peace and quiet you need for true rejuvenation.

The Life-Changing Magic of a Tidy Room

What does a clean bedroom have to do with good sleep? Everything.

Clutter in your bedroom can negatively affect your ability to rest. Having a messy space draws your attention, draining your energy as you fixate on misplaced items. Even if you're not the type to actively dwell on messiness, a chaotic environment influences the production of the stress hormone cortisol. When your cortisol levels rise, it's much more difficult to surrender into deep rest.

If "Messy" is your middle name, you don't need to change everything about yourself and your habits. Just make it a weekly priority to clean and organize your room. If it helps you to think of your bedroom as a sacred sleep chamber, please do. A tidy bedroom allows a mind to rest— and a rested mind allows your body to sleep.

So here are a few tips to start with:

* Don't leave piles of dirty clothes on the ground! Keep a laundry hamper in another room, if possible, and have a dedicated space for clothes that you intend to rewear.

* Change your sheets once a week. This will help keep your room dust- and allergen-free.

* Make your bed every morning! This instantly improves the look of your room and will give you a

feeling of satisfaction. Plus, there's nothing like slip-ping into a properly made bed at night.

* Adopt a no-clutter policy in the bedroom by keeping your dressers and nightstands free of tchotchkes. If you have devices that can live in another room, we encourage you to move them out.

Write It and Forget It

Even if you have a wonderful sleep routine and go to bed on time, it's hard to combat a mind that spins out of control whenever it's at rest. A racing mind continuously comes up with things to do, people to reach out to, events to remember, groceries to buy, and on and on. This is especially true if you're not taking breaks throughout the day to let your mind recover; it'll save everything up for bedtime.

Letting go of the day and surrendering to heaviness takes practice. If you have a mind that tends to race at night, consider writing a to-do list before bed as part of your evening ritual.

If you're particularly prone to anxiety, keep a journal next to your bed for those nights when your head won't stop spinning, so that you can quickly jot down your thoughts. The physical act of writing things down can provide instant relief. Don't try to organize your thoughts in a coherent way—and certainly don't get up to open your day planner, email, or calendar! This exercise is all about relief, not achievement. If you're really worried you'll forget something, you can always look back at your journal the next day.

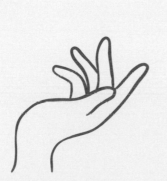

WHAT ARE YOUR MOST COMMON THOUGHTS
WHEN YOUR MIND RACES AT NIGHT?
DO YOU SEE A PATTERN IN THESE THOUGHTS?

IS THERE ANYTHING YOU CAN DO BEFORE BEDTIME THAT WILL HELP YOU FEEL MORE PREPARED FOR THE NEXT DAY?

No More Sheep

When you were a little kid, a grown-up in your life probably told you to imagine sheep jumping over a fence and to count them until you fell asleep. It's a cute idea, but spoiler alert: counting sheep doesn't really work! The technique isn't harmful but it doesn't help you combat intrusive thoughts, whether they be about something you said in a meeting that day or at a party three years ago.

A more modern approach, with a higher degree of success, is the visualization method. This allows you to distract yourself from unwanted thoughts with more in-depth immersive imagery, which will allow you to lapse into a state of restfulness. It's simple and highly effective, and it costs nothing.

* Imagine yourself in a peaceful place that feels right for you. A general nature setting, like mountains, woods, or the beach, will give you plenty of space to mentally roam.

* Engage all five senses. What do you hear, see, smell, taste, and feel?

* Make this scene come to life as much as possible. Think of plants, flowers, animals, the weather— whatever you can conjure.

* Keep envisioning the peaceful setting and everything in it until you find yourself drifting off.

If you miss the sheep, you can always add them to your scene!

USING THE VISUALIZATION METHOD, IMAGINE A
NATURAL SCENE THAT YOU CAN REVISIT AT NIGHTTIME.
JOT DOWN AS MANY DETAILS AS POSSIBLE!

Evening
Rituals

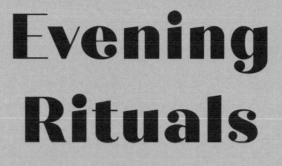

While this entire book contains tips and tricks that you can integrate into your sleep routine, in this chapter we want to focus solely on effective rituals and techniques that will help you deal with excess wind (which leads to overthinking) and a lack of earth (which prevents you from achieving peace).

The goal here is to redirect your inner winds and find inner peace. We'll also discuss when and how often you should perform these rituals and techniques so you can use your time most effectively. You don't need to incorporate all of them—just try a few that speak to you.

Breathe Yourself into Balance

As yoga practitioners, we often talk about the different energy channels that run through our bodies. Two of the biggest channels begin in your nostrils. The right nostril is associated with solar energy; it's expressive, hot, and focused outward. The left nostril is associated with lunar energy; it's intuitive, cool, and focused inward.

To bring both of these energies together in perfect balance, you can do a breath exercise called alternate nostril breathing. This technique is very calming and an excellent way to soothe your scattered mind at the end of the day.

Steps for alternate nostril breathing:

1. Sit in a comfortable position, with your spine elongated and your shoulders relaxed.

2. Gently close your right nostril with your right thumb. Inhale through your left nostril and then close it with your right pinky.

3. Remove your right thumb from your right nostril and exhale slowly through the right nostril.

4. Keep the right nostril open, inhale, then close it.

5. Open your left nostril and exhale slowly. This is one cycle.

6. Repeat for 3 to 5 minutes.

Do this daily in the evening.

The Yogic Power Nap

Even if you do everything right, there are going to be nights when you don't get enough sleep. This is especially true during high-stress times. You might be inclined to power through the next day with coffee and energy drinks but this can wreak havoc on your body and will lose its effectiveness over time.

A truly refreshing practice that will help you get through the rest of your day—and treat your nervous system more gently than caffeine—is yoga nidra. In yoga nidra, you use guided meditation to fall into a state of deep relaxation, somewhere in the space between wakefulness and sleep.

The best way to master this technique is by practicing with a certified yoga instructor. However, there are plenty of sleep and meditation apps available that work well too; just be sure to use a guided meditation meant for achieving deep relaxation.

Simply lie on the floor, a couch, or a bed while the instructor (virtual or in person) leads you through exercises meant to stimulate different brainwaves. This is a highly effective way to reap the benefits of deep rest without feeling sluggish afterward, which is an unfortunate side effect of a normal afternoon nap.

When you practice yoga nidra, make sure you set an alarm—you're at high risk for falling asleep! We recommend doing it on days when you haven't gotten enough sleep, though if you're prone to fatigue you can use it to manage your energy on a daily basis.

Zzz

Zzz

Zzz

Three-Stage Breathing

Most of us take shallow breaths, especially when we're busy or stressed out, which further exacerbates our stress. One of the fastest ways to achieve instant relaxation is by using the full capacity of your lungs. Taking long, slow, and full breaths activates your parasympathetic nervous system, which regulates anxiety and stress hormones in your body.

First, let's go over the three positions of three-stage breathing:

1   Lie on your back and place both of your hands on your lower belly, below your navel. Breathe normally. Notice your breath here. Maintain this position for about two minutes.

2   Slide your hands up so they're resting on the side of your ribs. Feel the expansion and softening of your ribcage. Maintain this position for about two minutes.

3   Slide your hands up farther so they're resting on your chest, beneath your collarbones. Feel the subtle movement of your breath. Maintain this position for about two minutes.

Now, let's incorporate these movements into your breathing cycle:

1   Slide your hands to your lower belly again and exhale fully. Inhale until you feel like your lungs are one-third full and hold that breath. Slide your hands to the side of your ribs and inhale until your lungs are two-thirds full and hold it. Slide your hands up to your chest and inhale the last third, ensuring your lungs are completely full, and hold it in.

2   Now *exhale* and slide your hands back down to the lower belly.

Repeat this for at least five cycles during moments of high stress.

Say a Little Prayer

Prayer doesn't belong just to the religious. When you feel like you're carrying the weight of the world on your shoulders, it can be helpful to adopt some perspective. It can be extremely freeing to acknowledge our place in the universe, to realize that we are a small part of the whole and that our actions aren't going to shake the sun, moon, and stars out of the sky.

When the trivial details of life are keeping you up at night, take a moment to say a prayer. You don't need to think of a specific recipient or give this nebulous entity a name; just focus on feeling humility and gratitude for the good things in life. This will ground you during periods of stress and better prepare you to accept the heaviness of sleep when the time comes.

Give Thanks

If the concept of prayer—even of the cosmic variety—is uncomfortable for you but you still want to reap its benefits, consider ending your day with gratitude.

Gratitude is a great way to combat common types of intrusive thoughts, including fixating on your fears and failures. Failures, in particular, have a way of replaying over and over in our heads. Working through these moments in therapy can help you change how you feel about these events and learn from your mistakes, but dwelling on them before bed will only leave you staring at the ceiling in regret.

The things you think about before bed have a major influence on what your subconscious mind focuses on during the night. To help change the narrative of your dreams, end your day with gratitude by mentally listing three things you're grateful for.

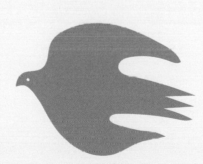

WHAT ARE YOU MOST GRATEFUL FOR?

WHAT GIVES YOU COMFORT WHEN THINGS AREN'T GOING WELL?

Read Your Way
to Relaxation

Books are a wonderful way to make you feel grounded and safe at the end of the day. Stories can remind you of thoughts, feelings, and truths you might've forgotten—or have yet to discover. They're also an effective distraction from intrusive thoughts and a great way to improve your cognitive function overall.

We love books about spirituality by authors who seem to have a direct line to the universe, but there's nothing wrong with a romance, thriller, or horror novel if that's more your speed! If you have trouble getting into books, consider joining a book club for extra motivation. You can look forward to the discussion—and the snacks!

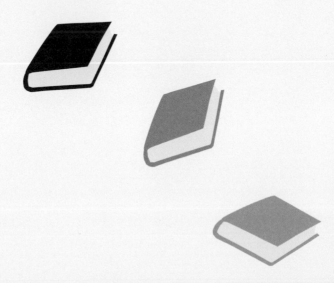

MAKE A LIST OF ALL THE BOOKS YOU'D LIKE TO READ
IN THE NEXT MONTH AS YOU WORK ON IMPROVING
YOUR SLEEP HYGIENE. NOTE WHAT EXCITES YOU
ABOUT THESE BOOKS!

Healing Stones

Crystals are more than beautiful objects—they're tools for connecting you to the earth. The element of earth is heavy, dense, stable, and slow. These are the qualities we're trying to achieve as we prepare for sleep. Read those four words a few times and you might even start to feel sleepy!

Earth is composed of thousands of minerals and each one carries different properties. While crystals are not scientifically proven to help you fall asleep, placing some next to your bed or holding a stone while you doze off is a nice way to invoke the element of earth and invite those heavy, dense, stable, and slow vibes into your evening.

We recommend these three crystals, each of which has properties that encourage relaxation and renewal:

* Rose quartz: This is the stone of love. It has a soothing and calming effect and is said to bring pleasant dreams.

* Amethyst: This stone brings protection and aligns you with divine wisdom.

* Moonstone: It's in the name! Moonstone carries the energy of the new moon, which stands for new beginnings.

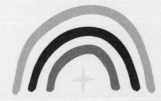

Bed Buddha

I don't have time for meditation.

I'm not good at meditation.

If one of these statements has ever come out of your mouth, let us change your mind.

First things first: Meditation is not about sitting still for an hour and thinking of nothing. Meditation can be as short as one minute long. It has a greater impact when practiced for longer periods, but starting with five, ten, or fifteen minutes is still excellent.

Meditation is not about *not* thinking—it's about catching yourself in the act of thinking. Instead of being carried away by the story you're telling yourself, meditation guides you back to the present moment by focusing on your breath. It's impossible to stop the formation of thoughts; the goal is to let those thoughts go as they arrive.

If you spend fifteen minutes thinking, that doesn't mean your meditation was unsuccessful. Your conclusion could be that your mind is very busy today. With that knowledge, you can help yourself by setting aside extra time before bed to clear your head. You can use this time to write down your thoughts, drink a cup of chamomile tea, or do any of the rituals and techniques described in this section.

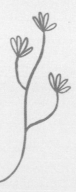

WHICH RITUALS AND TECHNIQUES FROM THIS SECTION SPEAK TO YOU THE MOST?

WHAT DOES YOUR IDEAL EVENING ROUTINE
LOOK LIKE NOW?

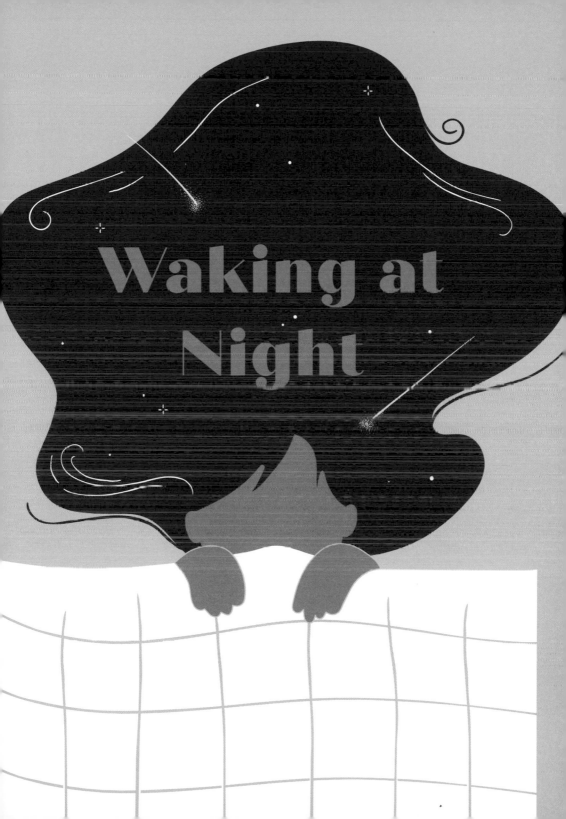

There are two categories of sleep issues. The first one is trouble falling asleep. The second is waking up in the middle of the night. You can suffer from one, the other, or both at the same time.

Waking up in the middle of the night can have several causes. One thing's for sure: it's no fun.

What we want to tell you is that there's no reason to panic. Remember, in the dark, everything seems much worse than it actually is; you literally and figuratively can't see clearly. Trust that everything will get better when the sun comes up—and that a few nights of bad sleep is manageable.

We're here to help you fall back asleep, or at least to keep you company in the dark.

Keep It Cool

If you regularly wake up between midnight and 2 a.m., this could indicate that your fire element is too strong. A too-strong fire element can express itself through literal heat—some sleepers run hot and tend to sweat throughout the night—but it can also manifest as a tendency to mentally loop through to-do lists and imagine arguments with people you're not getting along with.

There are several ways to turn down the heat on your midnight flame:

* Jot down any conflicts or points of tension you're feeling before you go to sleep.

* Reduce the temperature in your bedroom or open a window.

* Wear light pajamas—or go naked if you can!

* Dress your bed with season-appropriate bedding. Linen and percale are great for hot sleepers.

* Do a meditation focused on loving kindness before bed or in the middle of the night so you can fall back to sleep.

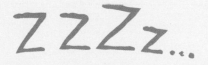

Calm Your Winds

If you regularly wake up after 2 a.m., this could indicate that your wind and space elements are too strong. Such a condition can express itself as waking up fearful and feeling ungrounded, but it can also manifest as an overactive mind that's anxious about the future.

There are several ways to calm your wind and space elements:

* Jot down your main anxieties shortly before you go to sleep.

* Sleep with a heavy or weighted blanket.

* Drink a soothing, warm drink before bed.

* Get yourself something to cuddle with! Another human, a pet, or a big teddy bear are all acceptable.

* Practice three-stage breathing.

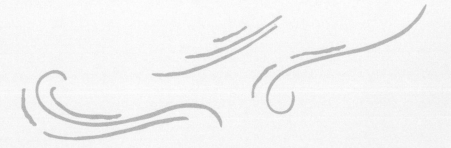

DO YOU STRUGGLE WITH HIGH FIRE OR STRONG WIND?
WHAT STEPS CAN YOU TAKE TO REBALANCE YOURSELF?

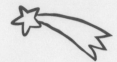

Banish Your Nightmares

Do you ever suddenly wake up from a dream scared, sweaty, disoriented, and with a racing heart? Chances are you just had a nightmare. Nightmares aren't the sweetest experience to wake up from—and it can be a challenge to fall back asleep after you have one. A particularly bad nightmare can even haunt you throughout the next day.

One of the most common triggers of nightmares is stress—of both the conscious and unconscious variety. When we're exposed to a lot of stress during the day, we carry that tension into our dreams. Watching, reading, and imagining scary things right before bed are also common triggers, especially if you're not a horror fan.

If you're prone to nightmares, we highly recommend swapping thrillers for comedies if you watch TV or read a book as part of your evening ritual.

If you're chronically stressed, we recommend starting your wind-down process as early in the evening as possible and focusing on relaxation for the last couple hours of your day. This might seem like a luxury to those who consider themselves constantly busy and overscheduled, but it's the most important thing you can do for yourself. If you're unwilling to make changes, it's almost impossible to break the chronic stress cycle. Evaluate your evening activities, be honest about what you can let go of, and prioritize relaxation the same way you would an important family or work task. Your ability to manage the things that are stressing you out will be even stronger if you get some good sleep.

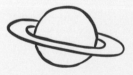

Guilt-Free Rest

We know we need to *sleep* every day, but did you know we also need to *rest* every day?

Rest and sleep are two sides of the same coin. Being rested and relaxed is the ideal condition for good sleep. If you find it difficult to take breaks throughout the day, chances are you have difficulty falling and staying asleep.

We live in a world where being successful and staying busy are highly valued. The less free time we have in our calendars, the better we're doing. We have to be on top of our game, always. Practicing yoga nidra or doing a legs up session in the afternoon might be anathema to you at first, and you might worry that others will judge you for being lazy or self-indulgent.

Think of it this way; we eat when we're hungry, we drink when we're thirsty, and we go to the bathroom when we need to pee or poop. Some of us postpone these natural urges but there's only so long you can go with an empty stomach or full bladder.

When we're tired, we completely fight the impulse to rest. We drink a cup of coffee or eat an energy bar—and we make this a habit that lasts years, maybe even a whole lifetime. But whether society agrees or not, this is unnatural and will throw your body out of whack in the form of chronic illnesses, mental health issues, and more.

Invest in guilt-free rest. Let's listen to our bodies without shame.

Trust Yourself

You look at the clock. The number frightens you. Only four more hours before your alarm goes off.

If you suffer from sleeplessness, the clock might actually contribute to your problems. When we count hours of sleep, we get anxious if the number doesn't meet our ideal amount of sleep—which keeps us awake and prevents us from getting as much rest as we possibly can.

Trust yourself! When you wake up in the middle of the night, don't look at the clock. Let the situation be just as it is. Try to relax. Notice your breath. Maybe do a yoga nidra practice. But don't worry about the number of hours. It's okay. You are okay.

HOW WILL YOU IMPLEMENT PERIODS
OF RELAXATION INTO YOUR DAY?

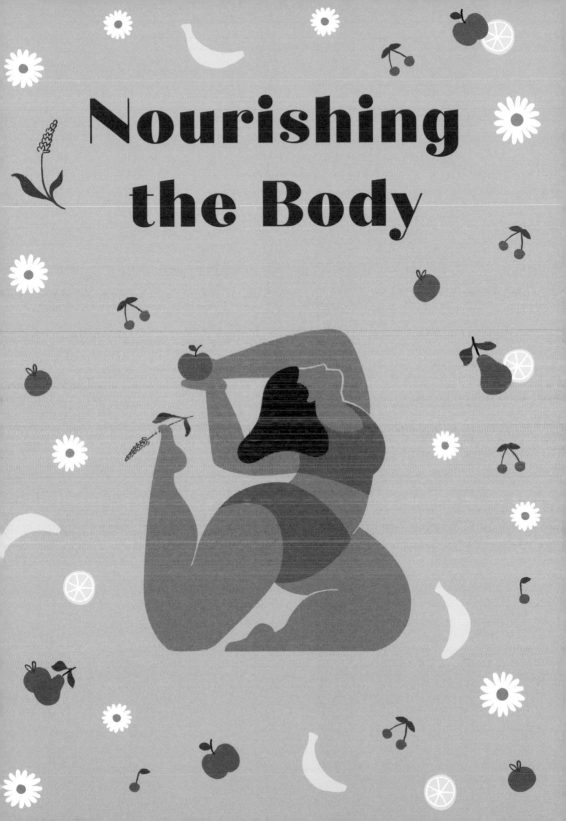

Nourishing the Body

Your body and mind are intimately connected to each other. What happens to your body has an impact on your mental health, and your mental health impacts how your body feels. This is why diet is so important. If you eat nourishing foods, your body will be at ease and your mind will be able to relax more easily.

Try not to assign moral value to foods. A holistic healthcare approach focuses on the energy that different foods supply. If you struggle with sleeplessness, use the recipes in this section to improve your digestive health—and set yourself up for bedtime success.

A Word About Eating in the Evening

If you adopt a holistic healthcare approach, the evening (from about 6 p.m. to 10 p.m.) should be dedicated to slowing down. Our digestive fire naturally cools at this time to prepare our bodies and minds for rest and sleep. However, in many cultures and families, dinner is a late-evening affair—and late-night snacking is common. This means we have to spend our energy digesting food rather than digesting thoughts. If you overeat or indulge in a late-night snack on top of it all, you may go to bed feeling uncomfortable from feelings of fullness, acid reflux, heartburn, or a mix of all three.

If you regularly wake up feeling like you've been hit by a truck, it's time to check your eating habits. If you're looking for healthy snacks that will help you sleep better, try some of the recipes over the next few pages!

WHAT ARE YOUR EVENING EATING HABITS?

IF YOU EAT A LATE-NIGHT SNACK REGULARLY, HOW DOES IT MAKE YOU FEEL?

Peaceful Herbs

If you have trouble catching zzz's, you can turn to a few herbal remedies. The following are known in Ayurveda for soothing the nervous system and helping you relax.

If you have questions about the impact of these herbs, especially if you're pregnant or nursing, or if you'll be ingesting them in dietary supplement form, please consult your doctor. For sleep purposes, we generally suggest ingesting them in tea form or mixing them into a warm beverage.

* Lavender: The smell of this flower alone can have an immediate calming effect, but drinking it in tea form is even more effective. If you have a lavender body or linen spray, mist it over your pillow before you go to sleep.

* Chamomile: This flower relieves stress and anxiety and is especially popular in tea form.

* Valerian: This plant reduces sleep latency, or the time needed to fall asleep once you lie down, and is great for insomniacs. This is commonly taken in dietary supplement form but the root can also be steeped into a tea.

* Nutmeg: This spice contains trimyristin, which relaxes the body. Incorporate it into your evening meal or sprinkle it into a warm beverage.

* Cinnamon: This spice relaxes tense muscles. Sprinkle it into a warm beverage.

* Ashwagandha: This medicinal herb is often taken in a tonic or as a dietary supplement to relieve long-term stress. It is known to improve energy and cognition.

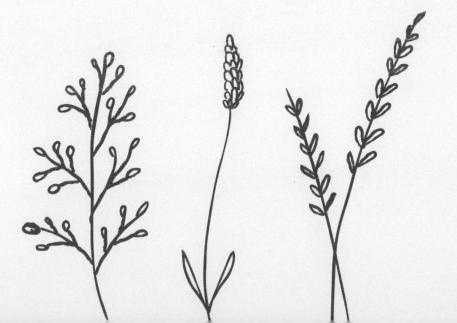

Sleep-Promoting Elixir

This elixir is perfect during the autumn and winter months when it's cold outside. Milk and dates are a magical combination and nourishing for the nervous system. Add a few spices and you have yourself an amazing and delicious evening drink.

INGREDIENTS

* 1 cup organic whole milk or almond milk

* 1 Medjool date, pitted

* Pinch of ground nutmeg

* ½ teaspoon ashwagandha powder (optional)

Blend the milk and date in a blender until smooth. Pour the mixture into a saucepan and heat gently. Add nutmeg and ashwagandha if using, stir, and serve.

Apple Cider Vinegar and Honey

This remedy sounds rather intense but the combination of these two power ingredients will help you get some shut-eye when you need it most. Apple cider vinegar contains vitamins and minerals that promote relaxation and help your body produce sleep hormones. Raw organic honey has been used throughout history to promote better sleep and relaxation.

INGREDIENTS

* 1 cup warm water

* ½ tablespoon apple cider vinegar, or more to taste

* ½–1 tablespoon raw organic honey, to taste

Mix all ingredients and pour into a mug. We suggest starting with ½ tablespoon of apple cider vinegar and gradually working your way up to 1 tablespoon as your palate gets acclimated to it over time.

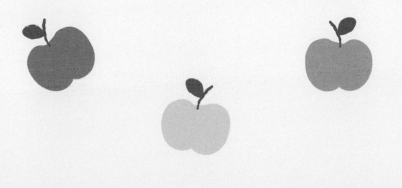

Bananas

You can find this tropical fruit in kitchens around the world. It can be eaten alone as a simple snack or folded into pancake batter, mashed into banana bread batter, sliced over ice cream, blended into smoothies …the list goes on! Bananas help alleviate muscle cramps, sleeplessness, and stress by enhancing melatonin and serotonin production and lowering your blood pressure.

BANANA SMOOTHIE

INGREDIENTS

* 1 banana

* 1 cup almond milk

* 1 teaspoon honey

* Pinch each of ground cinnamon and ground nutmeg

Mix all the ingredients in a blender until smooth. You can warm the blended drink a little to induce sleep.

VEGAN BANANA BREAD

If a smoothie isn't your choice of nighttime remedy, you can opt for this super-healthy version of banana bread. It's grounding, nourishing, yummy, and filled with ingredients that encourage deep sleep.

INGREDIENTS

* 4 ripe bananas (the riper, the better)

* 4 to 8 Medjool dates, to taste

* ¼ cup coconut flour

* 1 cup oat flour

* 2 tablespoons poppy seeds

* 1 teaspoon baking powder

* 1 teaspoon ground cinnamon

* ½ teaspoon ground nutmeg

* Pinch of salt

* 1 cup plant-based milk

* 1 teaspoon baking soda

* 1 tablespoon apple cider vinegar

1. Preheat the oven to 350 degrees Fahrenheit. Grease a standard loaf pan (8½ inches x 4½ inches x 2½ inches) and line it with parchment paper.

2. In a large bowl, mash the bananas and dates with a fork.

3. In a medium bowl, whisk together all the dry ingredients except the baking soda. Add mixture to mashed bananas and dates.

4. Stir in the milk. The mixture should form a thick batter.

5. In a small bowl, combine the baking soda and apple cider vinegar. You'll notice it will start to foam. This is a good thing! Add the foamy mixture to the batter.

6. Pour the batter into the prepared loaf pan and bake for 40–45 minutes. When a knife or toothpick inserted in the center of the loaf comes out clean, the bread is done.

7. Let the banana bread cool before serving!

TART CHERRY SMOOTHIE

Cherries, especially tart cherries, naturally contain melatonin. Drink this a couple of hours before bed!

INGREDIENTS

* 1 banana

* ½ cup tart cherry juice

* ½ cup almond milk

* Pinch of ground nutmeg

Mix everything in a blender and enjoy!

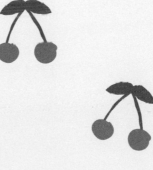

HOW DO YOU WANT TO FEEL AFTER YOU EAT?

ARE THERE FOODS THAT HELP YOU ACHIEVE THAT FEELING? DO ANY OF THE FOODS MENTIONED IN THIS SECTION APPEAL TO YOU?

Sleep Saboteurs

We're surrounded by temptations that make us feel good when we indulge in them but regretful when it's time to go to bed. Some are obvious—a bag of chips or a glass of wine right before you turn out the lights. Others might be less obvious—including a cup of coffee you drink in the morning. We'll tell you what to avoid and what to embrace, but keep in mind that it's up to you to decide what's best for you. We think it's okay to indulge once in a while, but we encourage you to be mindful about the connection between common sleep saboteurs and your overall health. Stay attuned to your body; it knows your limits.

Processed Foods

Processed foods are a common pitfall. We know that inhaling a bag of potato chips will make us feel sluggish, but what about that box of organic whole wheat crackers? And that frozen vegan pizza? How about those convenient, fresh-looking ready-to-eat meals at your local grocery store that you can quickly pop into the microwave?

We're sorry to tell you this but if it comes packaged or canned, it likely contains some form of additives or preservatives, as well as too much salt and saturated fat. Oftentimes, there's not enough nutrition in these foods to balance their downsides. Even processed food that's marketed as healthy is never as healthy as fresh, whole foods.

These foods might satisfy our cravings but they do not please our bodies. Our bodies are looking for prana, or life energy. Foods with low nutritional value that are hard to digest offer the opposite of prana; they make our bodies expend energy so that we are sluggish and tired when we should feel energized. They wreak havoc on our digestive systems and have a direct impact on the quality of our sleep.

Your body will be happiest if you nourish yourself with whole grains, fruits, and veggies—but we also understand that you're not a robot that can be programmed to automatically like these foods, and you don't necessarily have the time to prepare healthy meals with these foods three times a day.

We like to follow the 80/20 rule: we're responsible eaters 80 percent of the time, which gives us plenty of space for treats and convenience eating when we're pressed for time. By adhering to the 80/20 rule, your emotional cravings will be fulfilled and your body will reward you with a good night's sleep.

Delicious Substitutes for Coffee

Coffee substitutes? I think I'll skip this chapter!

We can hear you from here—and we understand! Coffee is sacred for many of us, especially after a rough night. More than that, the ritual of making coffee in the morning can ground you (no pun intended) before you plunge into your hectic day.

Coffee has some notable health benefits but it's also easy to abuse—and most coffee-drinkers do just that. If you drink multiple cups a day, you're overstimulating your mind, which can set you on edge and make you anxious. Over time, coffee can have the opposite of its desired effect: your body relies on caffeine instead of natural energy and tires more easily, leading to fatigue and burnout.

Fortunately there a few ways to raise your energy levels in a meaningful way without overstimulating your nerves. We like:

* Golden milk made with turmeric

* Hot chocolate from raw cacao

* Herbal tea

* Rooibos tea

* Root grain coffee

No to Nightcaps

A glass of wine seems like the perfect way to help you fall asleep more easily . . . and it is! The downside is that it affects the quality of your sleep, especially during the REM stage of your sleep cycle. During REM sleep, you process all your mental impressions of the day. It's highly restorative and crucial for rebuilding energy. When this stage is disrupted by tossing and turning or dehydration, you might feel drowsy and unable to concentrate the next day.

Still hesitant to give up your nightcap? Have a look at these figures from a 2018 Finnish study that assessed the impact of alcohol intake on the autonomic nervous system.

* Low alcohol intake reduces sleep quality by 9.3 percent.

* Moderate alcohol intake reduces sleep quality by 24 percent.

* Heavy alcohol intake reduces sleep quality by 40 percent.

Here's what you can do if you don't want to completely give up this saboteur:

* Don't drink alcohol within 3 hours of bedtime.

* Stay hydrated.

* Have your drink with a meal.

Blame It on the Moon

The moon is Earth's scapegoat. If there's a spike in crime, or if you're more prone to mood swings and sleepless nights at a certain time of the month, folk wisdom tells you to blame it on the moon.

In the case of crime and mood swings, these assertions aren't scientific—but in the case of sleep, it's okay to blame the moon a little bit!

Our bodies naturally follow a circadian rhythm—a twenty-four-hour cycle that dictates behaviors like sleeping. As our environment changes, we change. When the moon is full, there's naturally more light in the sky, which influences our melatonin levels. This has an impact on our ability to fall and stay asleep.

Whether or not the moon is affecting you in particular, set aside the days leading up to the full moon for some extra relaxation. Pamper yourself with herbal tea, a good book, and a bath in the evening. If this forces you to cancel some plans, just blame it on the moon.

WHAT ARE YOUR MAIN SLEEP SABOTEURS?
WHAT ARE YOUR STRATEGIES FOR ELIMINATING
OR REPLACING THEM?

Rest to Digest

If you spend your whole day in front of cell phones, computers, and TV screens, or live in a city full of skyscrapers and largely empty of trees, it's important to be mindful of how your circumstances might be impacting your mental and emotional health.

Our bodies weren't meant to be plugged in to the internet all day, and yet many of us live like this day after day, year after year. This can drain your energy, and it's also a tough way to treat your brain. If your brain is checked out, it's going to have a tough time processing experiences and emotions and finding joy and relaxation in rituals as simple as a warm foot bath.

Relaxation requires mental participation and engagement with the present. If you regularly feel like your brain isn't in your body, it's going to be hard for you to relax—and to fall and stay asleep.

But don't worry. We have a few last tips for you before we let you go.

Comforting Words

If you were afraid of the dark as a child, your mom, dad, or caretaker might've held you in their arms and told you everything was okay—that there were no monsters in the closet or under the bed, that you were safe, and that they would protect you if anything were to happen. Do you remember that feeling of warmth and comfort?

You can give that feeling to yourself by allowing your higher self to take care of your little self. Instead of letting your worries take over, let your higher self rise and repeat some positive affirmations. Breaking negative thought patterns is difficult but remember: the child within you needs a grown-up to say something comforting every once in a while. Thankfully, that grown-up lives within you, too.

Affirmations are a very personal practice, but try out a few of these and see if they resonate with you.

* I am safe, I am loved, all is well.

* I deserve deep, restorative sleep.

* Thank you, universe, for taking care of me.

* I trust the natural cycles of the universe.

* I let go and surrender to sleep.

The Art of Resting

Most of us aren't great at resting—but that's okay! It's hard stuff and we don't always have good examples in our lives to follow.

If you find yourself constantly distracting yourself, staying busy, and resisting sleep, it's likely that you're trying to avoid yourself. We completely understand; it can be scary to spend time alone with your mind. However, the only way to truly restore yourself is to be alone with yourself without distractions so your mind can truly rest. Staying busy with projects and watching a few YouTube videos aren't going to cut it.

Resting should be in our agenda every day. The good news is that it can be as short as ten minutes and requires little to nothing.

Here are a few things you can do in those ten minutes.

1   Lie down on your sofa with your eyes closed. Notice your breath, feel your body, and listen to the sounds coming and going. Be present in the here and now.

2   Go outside and touch a tree, observe a flower, or notice the movements of an insect. Let nature guide you.

3   Drink a cup of tea. Savor each sip.

4   Eat a piece of fruit. Really taste it. Chew slowly. Notice the texture. Feel it nourishing your body.

5   Give yourself permission to be alone and do nothing.

Cuddle Time

The most loving way to spend more time in dreamland is to snuggle up with a partner or loved one. Cuddling relieves stress and gives both of you instant comfort. Submitting to a warm embrace will create feelings of being protected and held—great ingredients for a peaceful sleep.

Your cuddle partner does not need to be a person! Cats, dogs, and teddy bears are okay too. Happy cuddling!

WHICH RITUALS, TECHNIQUES, AND PRACTICES FROM
THIS BOOK DO YOU MOST WANT TO TRY AS YOU HEAD
INTO YOUR 21 DAYS OF GOOD SLEEP?

WHAT DO YOU NEED TO DO TO INCORPORATE THESE INTO YOUR DAILY LIFE?

21 Days of Good Sleep

We hope that reading this book was a great experience and will set you on a journey toward the best sleep of your life! Now that you know what lifestyle adjustments you want to make, use the next three weeks to try them out and track their impact on your sleep. Keep the adjustments that are working for you and let go of the ones that aren't. Happy sleeping!

Week Two

	MONDAY	TUESDAY	WEDNESDAY
TIME OF LAST MEAL			
TIME OF LAST CAFFEINE INTAKE			
TIME OF LAST ALCOHOL INTAKE			
TIME OF LAST WATER INTAKE			
SLEEP RITUALS			
SLEEP AIDS TAKEN			
TIME IN BED			
TIME YOU FELL ASLEEP			
DID YOU WAKE DURING THE NIGHT? (Y/N)			
MINUTES AWAKE			
NUMBER OF BATHROOM VISITS			
FINAL WAKE-UP TIME			
NIGHTMARES (Y/N)			
TOTAL HOURS OF SLEEP			
RESTED FEELING (1-10)			

THURSDAY	FRIDAY	SATURDAY	SUNDAY

Reflections on Week Two:

WHAT WORKED?
WHAT DIDN'T WORK?
WHAT ADJUSTMENTS DO I NEED TO MAKE?

Week Three

	MONDAY	TUESDAY	WEDNESDAY
TIME OF LAST MEAL			
TIME OF LAST CAFFEINE INTAKE			
TIME OF LAST ALCOHOL INTAKE			
TIME OF LAST WATER INTAKE			
SLEEP RITUALS			
SLEEP AIDS TAKEN			
TIME IN BED			
TIME YOU FELL ASLEEP			
DID YOU WAKE DURING THE NIGHT? (Y/N)			
MINUTES AWAKE			
NUMBER OF BATHROOM VISITS			
FINAL WAKE-UP TIME			
NIGHTMARES (Y/N)			
TOTAL HOURS OF SLEEP			
RESTED FEELING (1-10)			

THURSDAY	FRIDAY	SATURDAY	SUNDAY

Reflections on Week Three:

WHAT WORKED?

WHAT DIDN'T WORK?

WHAT ADJUSTMENTS DO I NEED TO MAKE?

118

Week Four

	MONDAY	TUESDAY	WEDNESDAY
TIME OF LAST MEAL			
TIME OF LAST CAFFEINE INTAKE			
TIME OF LAST ALCOHOL INTAKE			
TIME OF LAST WATER INTAKE			
SLEEP RITUALS			
SLEEP AIDS TAKEN			
TIME IN BED			
TIME YOU FELL ASLEEP			
DID YOU WAKE DURING THE NIGHT? (Y/N)			
MINUTES AWAKE			
NUMBER OF BATHROOM VISITS			
FINAL WAKE-UP TIME			
NIGHTMARES (Y/N)			
TOTAL HOURS OF SLEEP			
RESTED FEELING (1-10)			

THURSDAY	FRIDAY	SATURDAY	SUNDAY

Reflections on Week Four:

WHAT WORKED?
WHAT DIDN'T WORK?
WHAT ADJUSTMENTS DO I NEED TO MAKE?

Full Library of Congress Cataloging-in-Publication Data available upon request.

ISBN: 978-1-68369-333-8

Printed in China

Typeset in Greycliff, Larosa, and Quiche

Designed by Paige Graff
Production management by John J. McGurk

First published in Dutch by Kosmos Uitgevers, The Netherlands in 2022. Illustrations by Roel Steenbergen.

Quirk Books
215 Church Street
Philadelphia, PA 19106
quirkbooks.com

10 9 8 7 6 5 4 3 2 1